FREE OF
'INCURABLE'
CANCER

Susan Paton

FREE OF
'INCURABLE'
CANCER

Living in Overtime

Baraka
Books
Montréal

© Baraka Books

ISBN 978-1-77186-205-9 pbk; 978-1-77186-221-9 epub; 978-1-77186-222-6 pdf

Cover by Richard Carreau
Book Design by Folio infographie
Editing by Robin Philpot and Barbara Rudnicka
Illustrations by Jean-Pierre Dubreuil

Legal Deposit, 2nd quarter 2020
Bibliothèque et Archives nationales du Québec
Library and Archives Canada

Published by Baraka Books of Montreal; printed and bound in Quebec.

Trade Distribution & Returns
Canada – UTP Distribution: UTPdistribution.com

United States and world
Independent Publishers Group: IPGbook.com

We acknowledge the support from the Société de développement des entreprises culturelles (SODEC) and the Government of Quebec tax credit for book publishing administered by SODEC.

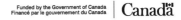

Contents

INTRODUCTION

Dear ———————,

I have not yet met you but when I heard of your cancer diagnosis, I knew I wanted to write to you. I have a sense of how you are feeling, although we all react differently upon hearing such news.

My ten-year journey with lymphoma has been terrifying, fascinating, instructive, humbling, difficult, and rewarding. My intent in sharing it with you is to help you find your path to hope and healing as others have done for me.

You may be surprised and unaccepting of some of my beliefs at first, but I simply invite you to consider possibilities and spend some time exploring them. Trust that a healthy curiosity can lead to some powerful insights.

Foremost, I suggest that you consider both the body and mind, as requiring healing. Illness can serve us by pointing towards unresolved emotional issues and beliefs.

We are constantly bathing in the product of our emotional state, both inside and outside of our body.

When illness strikes, our first, and usually only, reaction is to get a diagnosis and evaluate our medical treatment options. We focus on the physicality involved. But it is also vital to explore how our emotional history has contributed to—or caused—our current state of being unwell. We are more than a head and a body, so often seen as separate.

FALL 2009 – DISCOVERY

What the ....!

I am in the shower and suddenly feel a largish lump in my groin. Hmmmm.

Now lumps are never a reassuring thing to discover, but I decide to stay cool and not get too upset.

As I am already scheduled for my bi-annual mammogram at the breast clinic later this month, I plan to show this surprising new addition to my body to the oncologist there.

Yes, yes, I know as well as anyone, the breast is a bit far anatomically speaking from the groin, but I already have an appointment at that clinic, and I really like my doctor there.

So, several days later, while she is examining the top half, I show her the lump. She has many years of experience as an oncologist and I have great confidence in her. Since she wants me to have an ultrasound for my breasts, she laughingly announces that I can also have my lump scanned. No extra charge!

The ultrasound doctor checks me out, top and bottom, and even does a needle biopsy on my new-found lump. He says he sees no problems, but to come back in six weeks if it is still present.

This I find immensely reassuring and toast the good news with an evening glass of wine.

NERVOUSNESS

Over the next few days, however, I take quite a dislike to that little lump and decide to get it checked out by my family doctor. This is tricky as my family doc is in the process of retiring. I therefore decide to pay the big bucks and go to a private clinic (quickly) and see a doctor there who has been highly recommended.

While I describe the new-found lump situation to her, I carefully scrutinize her face. It is hard to tell if she thinks my situation is worrisome because she is totally poker-faced. But whether through concern or professionalism, she schedules me to have another ultrasound at her clinic the very next day. I can't quite decide if I think this is good news or not.

The following morning, I find myself with an older, really experienced ultrasound technician there. He is quite friendly as he says all seems in tip-top shape—even my liver (which is heartening, given my predilection for good wine). Then, I ask him specifically about the lump. He had not yet noticed it, as he was concentrated on my abdomen.

As he passes the wand back and forth, he gets super excited and suddenly proclaims he is sure I have lymphoma. He proudly points out to me certain oddly shaped cells (odd according to him—how would I know???). This is my very first time seeing my own cells of course. He describes in detail why this shape means lymphoma. He appears very pleased with himself for his rapid identification of the problem.

But I am stunned beyond words and just sit there staring at him. What am I to make of it all? Surely cancer cannot be so easily diagnosed? And who has ever received a cancer diagnosis directly from the ultrasound technician?

Finally, he is finished, and somehow I get dressed while mentally questioning his competence, not to mention his enthusiasm at sharing his findings.

I spend the rest of the evening trying to convince myself he should have retired years earlier.

It is such a bizarre event that I am worried, but not panicking. I also keep reminding myself that the results from the first ultrasound were negative.

Three days later, I return to my new family doctor for the results. I sit on the edge of my chair waiting for her to say that there has been some sort of mistake (and the ultrasound technician has been fired). She does not yet have his report in my file, so I wait another agonizing few minutes while she goes off to find it. Her reaction to his report (with the same poker-face), is to find the name and telephone number of a highly respected hematologist/oncologist in order to verify just what is going on. Not the reaction that I was looking for! She telephones the receptionist for this doctor, tells me I will be called back soon, and sends me quickly on my way.

A NEW WORLD

Thus begins my entry into a new and scary world with its own vocabulary, rules, and fears.

Unfortunately, the oncologist my doctor recommended is not accepting new patients, but his immensely kind assistant steers me to the right person who gets me an appointment that same week with another doctor on the oncology team. My sense of time is completely altered and I feel suspended in a state of febrile unreality.

A few days later, I manage to find the correct floor at the hospital, and the elevator doors open to bring me face to face with a very overcrowded waiting room. Standing room only, especially for those like me who look healthy. There is every type of personified fear to observe, and believe me, I am sure my own fear is palpable too. Some people are skeletal, others are bald, many look sad, several do not, and a few are very loud, while most whisper or are silent.

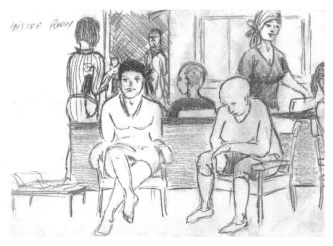

I quickly learn the drill—first the receptionist, next the vampires to have your blood drawn. These technicians are so effective; you don't even feel the needle going in! Then the little tubes of blood are sucked up to another floor for analysis and the results are on your doctor's screen within minutes. That is the efficient and quick part of the process, because afterwards, you wait and wait and wait to actually see the hematologist/oncologist.

Needless to say, I certainly do not want to be here and part of this!

My name is called, finally, and the whole process begins.

As this is a teaching hospital affiliated with a university, the first round of questions is with the resident, who is not much more relaxed looking than I. He is training in radiation oncology and seems a bit unsure what to ask me. Together we stumble through the process.

When the "real" doctor finally does come into the examining room, she looks exhausted, impatient, and is terse and abrupt. She asks me basically the same questions I have just answered with the resident, examines my lump and announces that she does not think it is cancer, but we must do a biopsy to confirm her evaluation. Hope surges through me and I am twenty pounds lighter!

My appointment with the surgeon for the biopsy is scheduled for January.

My exit from the hospital is as fast as possible while I attempt to maintain a semblance of calm.

MOMENTARY REPRIEVE

Shortly after that, I head out to Calgary for Christmas with my family, trying to be upbeat for myself as well as for the others.

One of my brothers-in-law is a doctor and a cancer survivor. He hypothesizes that I probably have some kind of infection I got from my cat. (Need I say he is a dog person?) The Siamese cat they once owned had the delightful habit of waking him by lying directly on his face. In retaliation, he became allergic which required a new home to be found for her.

I cling to his erudite explanation and mostly enjoy the holidays.

DIAGNOSIS

In mid-January, my sister—and number one support system—Anne comes to Montreal to accompany me for the biopsy operation. About one week earlier, I had already met with the surgeon—a super guy who explained all the details of the procedure. My anxiety levels are always much lower when someone takes the time to let me know exactly what will be happening.

Basically, this small operation only involves removing one lymph node from the groin area. Of course, it is always preferable to require an operation in another more public area of your body. Anyone—even medical professionals—staring intently at your groin for many minutes is disconcerting to say the least. But that darn lump had not consulted me about placement—or anything else in fact.

The operation is quick and easy with only a local anesthetic, which allows me to hear the surgeon teach his resident how to do beautiful stitches! I'm so glad things will be neatly sewn back in place. He kindly wishes me good luck as I exit the operating room. Something in the way he says it gives me pause, but then I shrug it off as needless worry.

Three weeks later, when I return to the oncologist for the results, I confidently expect to hear good news, and have managed to push back to the far corners of my mind the possibility of the worst.

It has not even occurred to me to ask one of my friends to accompany me.

After the usual lengthy wait, my name is finally called.

As soon as I sit down in the doctor's office, she immediately bluntly tells me that she was wrong and I do in fact have cancer and will require more tests. The preliminary diagnosis is Follicular Lymphoma.

There may be no easy way to give such news, but this is certainly incredibly expedient. I am with her for a maximum of ten minutes—it feels like two. There is no putting an arm on my hand or speaking reassuring words.

Everything is rushed and she attempts to hand me off to a nurse before she races off herself. Unfortunately, the nurse, very apologetic, is already booked to see someone else. All she has time for is to hand me a large book detailing the many different types of lymphoma.

I desperately want to get out of the hospital as quickly as possible and somehow find the proper elevator and stumble towards my car. Everything seems unreal and terrifying at the same time. I am not sure my ears work anymore. I seem to be inside a bubble.

I think of the old guy, the ultrasound technician, and have new-found respect for his amazingly accurate diagnosis. He had hit the nail on the head.

I stagger out of the hospital to find a parking ticket being placed on my car. I almost laugh. Somehow, it does not seem very important!

The first tears begin.

I manage to drive home without falling apart.

FEAR

Anne calls and having to tell her and say the very words make it all too scary. It is so tough to tell all my friends and family. To keep repeating that I have cancer is like pounding the nail of fear further and further into my gut. So I only speak to a very few and either e-mail the others or ask my sister to telephone them.

Then, of course, I read the section of the nurse's book on lymphoma that pertains to follicular lymphoma. Next I Google and start reading everything I can find online on this subject. Nothing I see is particularly optimistic, neither the treatments available, nor the outcomes. A cold hard ball of fear settles in my stomach.

For some as yet unexplained reason, I have a morbid, irrational fear of chemotherapy. The fact that many hundreds of thousands go through chemo every year does nothing to allay my anxiety. Guess what the only treatment option is? I panic every time I think about it and try to picture myself bald—not a pretty thought.

It seems stupefyingly trivial—even in the throes of my fear—to worry about being bald instead of being alive, but perhaps that is the only result I am able to cope with at this moment.

WHY?

Over the next weeks, as I try to understand and cope with what is going on, one thing becomes extremely clear to me. I never ask the question "Why me?" as in why should it be me who has cancer instead of someone else. But I cannot stop asking myself "*Why*?" There is no sense of guilt or personal responsibility for something I may have done wrong, only a deep conviction that there is a reason why this cancer has appeared.

After much reflection, I become absolutely convinced that my cancer was triggered by the break-up of a relationship about two years earlier. I had reacted so strongly to that event, and it had taken me a long while to get over it. I could see myself at that time feeling totally abandoned and at a loss. My reaction was completely out of line with my normal coping skills. I somehow *know* that this crisis, having deeply affected my emotional state and therefore my whole body, had brought on this illness. But I don't know what to do with this information as the damage is already done.

"BY THE WAY," MORE BAD NEWS

A few weeks later, my true-blue sister comes back to Montreal again to accompany me for the bone marrow biopsy. This is another test, done after a surgical biopsy to determine if there are cancer cells in the bone marrow. It is an exquisite form of torture that fortunately only lasts about ten minutes. My brother-in-law, who is very stoic, tells me that the pain he experienced with this test was severe and impossible to describe. So, I am feeling hugely nervous about the pain to come.

As we are awaiting the technician for this test, my oncologist very casually mentions that, in fact, my diagnosis has changed. She actually says "BY THE WAY, your diagnosis has been changed to Mantle Cell Lymphoma." Anne and I look agape at one another. Having no idea what that is—I know every horrid detail about the other one; I ask her what that means. Her reply is "*not good*." Now those are glad tidings!

She repeats that the initial diagnosis was preliminary, and that this one is final, based on the results provided from the lymph-node biopsy.

Anne and I are stunned at the casualness with which this information is delivered, and the timing, when I am already extremely anxious about the pain to come with the bone marrow biopsy.

The oncologist offers me an injection beforehand to reduce the pain, but does not really recommend it as she says it hurts as much as the actual biopsy. So, I decide to forego the injection—*very* bad advice from her and a worse decision of mine! The pain is excruciating for the short time it lasts. My sister says I levitated from the waist up during the procedure. Apparently, some people do not feel the level of agony I do, as pain is different for each person. Good for them because I truly would not wish this on anyone.

I do believe that lunch today will involve wine, but no problem, as my liver has been pronounced in good shape by that ever-so-accurate ultrasound tech.

Then back to the lymphoma book and the Internet to get details on this new "*not good*" diagnosis.

THE DIAGNOSIS WORSENS

That short biopsy agony is enough for "them" to determine that I do have cancer cells in my bone marrow. This then allows my doctor to define exactly the stage of my cancer. I learn that I am at stage 4b (not so good, as the best result starts at 1 and the end is at 4a). The more I find out about my situation, the worse it gets.

Basically, it appears that the medical profession knows very little about this particular disease. This type of lymphoma seems quite rare, and even more so in women. Also, there does not appear to be much mention of survival over the long haul—long being about five years.

Since, bizarrely, I do not have any other symptoms (this type of cancer is normally very aggressive and requires treatment immediately upon diagnosis), the option is "Watch and Wait."

I feel perfectly healthy and have no problems working and leading my life as usual, outside of the ever-present fear. Watch and wait suits me to a T because of my dread of chemo—the sole treatment on offer.

My wonderful friend Dana gets help from her compassionate colleagues in Boston and accompanies me to an appointment with the top Mantle Cell Lymphoma doctor there to get a second opinion. He is extremely professional and kind. They repeat the biopsy with tissue sent from my Montreal hospital and confirm the results. So, I cannot hope that there has been some error of diagnosis. But a visit with a fantastic friend, while under duress, is always immensely therapeutic. Speaking of which, I pour out to her at lunch the contents of my anxiety-filled soul and she listens and empathizes as always.

So, the good news is no poisoning my body for now, and the bad news is … the dark days begin.

WHAT IS IT ABOUT 3 A.M.?

I will not pretend that there are not many moments of total panic. Nights are often interminable and filled with the worst-case scenarios, which in fact concern suffering not death. Days are much more manageable. Just what is it about 3 a.m.?

My oncologist compounds this by announcing that this type of cancer is "*incurable*" and according to her statistics, my life expectancy is six years. Yikes! This of course makes me worry, and then I worry about wasting time worrying when I should be living to the hilt while I can.

Sleep is often beyond the possible except for a few hours filled with dreadful nightmares, usually involving treatment horrors.

Every twitch, small pain, imagined other lump is cause to descend into the jaws of terror. In fact, I think I basically live in a state of terror. Of course, some days are better than others; there are highs and lows. And my family and most fantastic group of friends do all they can.

DO SOMETHING

Several months after the diagnosis, I go to Paris to see my close friend Anik. She is a highly accomplished psychotherapist, a true friend, and is also very tuned in to alternative medicines.

As I am still in shock and unable to react or move forward, Anik shakes me and makes me understand that I have to *do something*, and that other options exist outside of our traditional Western medicine. And remember that Western medicine has nothing to offer me but a dismal scenario.

She has heard of a man in Chartres, a bio-chemist who has worked for many years in one of the top cancer hospitals in Paris. He says he can treat cancer with natural medicines.

So off we go. At least Chartres has a beautiful cathedral to discover if our visit is not helpful.

When we meet our bio-chemist in his run-down little office, we are somewhat stupefied by him. He is jovial, needs lots of personal reinforcement, and yet somehow convinces the two of us that I should take his herbal concoctions. As it is all natural and cannot harm me, plus I have no other options, I agree to take a six-month supply.

Our Western medical culture with its huge pharmacopeia has us believe that swallowing something will help. So I feel better just doing something! Watching and waiting can get wearisome. It make your feel ineffective.

We immediately baptize him "Professeur Tournesol" after the wonderful French storybook Tintin. I follow his regimen religiously, visiting him to change the formula every six months, based on his botanical knowledge and his piece of quartz dangling on a chain. I call the tinctures his "magic potions" and hardly ever miss a day, morning and evening.

Do I KNOW if they help me? No, I do not, but I can tell you that taking action and having someone give me hope are immensely positive. We all need a reason to hope and at this moment, he is mine. I will be forever grateful to him for that.

And of course, more so to my friend Anik for getting me started on my healing journey. Because now I do consider this a fascinating journey that will end up with me at a ripe old age.

SELF-HYPNOSIS

At a dinner party, an acquaintance—a cancer survivor himself—suggests I look into self-hypnosis. Of course, I immediately picture those TV shows where people suddenly start to imagine they are playing the tuba or some such ridiculous thing after the hypnotist has worked his magic.

He says how beneficial this has been for him and recommends a book.

Another friend suggests I find a good therapist to teach it to me, as it is not necessarily easy to learn on your own.

This idea of hypnosis appeals to me strongly.

When you are diagnosed with cancer, many people recommend various remedies, books, and self-help treatments out of kindness and concern. All I can say, based on my personal experience, is that for some unscientific reasons, certain options appeal to you, whereas others don't. I go with my gut, and feel it serves me well.

A psychologist friend whose strong code of ethics prevents him from working with me, as a personal friend, recommends another excellent therapist to teach me self-hypnosis.

Naturally, the reality of self-hypnosis is far removed from the tuba-playing of stage shows.

At first, I think I must not be "getting it" as nothing extraordinary is happening. But with reassurance from my inspiring therapist, I stop pushing myself and try to relax into non-goal-oriented openness.

I LOVE learning self-hypnosis, learning how to let my mind go into a deep, peaceful state.

During one of these sessions, I begin to experience some weird and wonderful moments. Once, I feel I am seeing my brain! I always come away feeling refreshed and renewed. It really is another form of meditation which is so powerful. During these sessions, I am without fear and fully alive in the moment—a welcome respite.

And now, I am able to use this fabulous tool anytime on my own.

A NEW ONCOLOGIST

I learn that my oncologist will be departing on maternity leave, and I choose another in the same department who has been recommended to me through friends.

What a difference in demeanour! I like his smiling, friendly approach. He is more aligned to my emotional needs. He is experienced and never utters a word that does not inspire hope. In short, he listens to me and adapts to my needs as much as possible. Also, he never infers that there is such a thing as "impossible" in medicine or in life.

Do doctors remember how important this is to their patients? Unfortunately, no, not all do.

A SURPRISE

Many months after my diagnosis, I awake early one morning and immediately feel something is different. I soon realize that for the first time, I feel no terror. I cannot recall a dream or any other reason for this to occur, but it is an incredible relief. I sense that I am doing all I can and now must let go. Of course, my fear does come back from time to time, but it is never as debilitating or overwhelming as before.

A MEDIUM

So, here I am going to France every six months to renew the magic potions (talk about a silver lining!).

In April 2012, Anik and I go to Bordeaux for a holiday week to celebrate her birthday after our visit to our mad "Professeur Tournesol."

She has heard of a medium in that area who comes highly recommended and thinks he may be able to provide some direction in my journey.

Luckily, I am quite open to this idea since there had been mediums used in my mother's family.

In fact, our family lore holds that two of my great-uncles discovered an iron ore mine in Atikokan in Northwestern Ontario because one of their long-deceased wives appeared in a dream and directed them to the correct site.

My Dad who was an engineer by training and a very pragmatic businessman had attended séances with my

Mom's uncles in his younger days and he had "seen" his father (who had died when my Dad was just sixteen).

My father explained the phenomenon this way: If you had told his grand-mother that one day she would sit in her living-room and see "live" singers on stage, say in London, in a box on her table, she would have been absolutely certain you were crazy.

My parents felt that we simply did not yet have the explanation for the ability of certain persons to "see" into the future.

I also believe that some people are able to tap into or pass beyond the time/space continuum in a different way than most of us. The bit of reading I have attempted in order to grasp a basic concept of Quantum physics seems to validate such an idea. So clearly this is a concept I am open to and at ease to deal with.

BERNARD

Upon meeting Bernard, he seems so much an "ordinary" guy that I am puzzled and unsure if he is qualified. Not that I thought I had any preconceived ideas of how a medium should look, but obviously "ordinary" does not compute. However, soon after he begins, I am amazed by his abilities.

I was already convinced that my illness was triggered by the extremely strong reaction I had to a failed relationship a couple of years before I was diagnosed. My emotions then were severe. I was depressed and could not seem to get over it and start to move on for close to a year. As I said before, I connected this reaction to the onset of my illness.

Bernard starts by asking me what I wish him to talk about, because otherwise he can go in many directions and thus possibly not answer my main concerns.

I name several subjects for discussion and slide in the topic of my health somewhere in the middle.

Now the only thing Bernard knows about me is that I am from Montreal. Before our meeting, he was given no information about me other than where and when I was born.

I am not on Facebook at this time, and "googling" me will produce no results.

And I do not inform him of my diagnosis, nor volunteer any other information. What's more, I show absolutely no exterior signs of ill-health—quite the contrary.

When he begins by asking me about a previous relationship that had not worked out and had left me feeling abandoned, I am listening hard. After some twenty minutes during which he advances totally relevant and factual comments about my life, I end up telling him of my recent diagnosis.

He says my illness was caused by my reaction to this failed relationship and recommends in no uncertain terms a book on his desk entitled *Métamédecine* by a Quebec author called Claudia Rainville. She is well known in Europe. He tells me she had cured herself of cancer and that I should consult her work and even try to see her if feasible.

According to Bernard, I will not be *dérangée* (bothered) by this illness and I should do some work on understanding why I developed it, possibly with a therapist and also on my own. A huge feeling of relief washes over me! It *is* possible that those dire predictions will not come to pass!

He feels the presence of my mother very strongly and says she is often with me and helping me. He says she was responsible for my fear suddenly leaving me earlier this year.

There is nothing odd or weird in the way Bernard discusses this. He is matter-of-fact in his approach. We meet in a small rather bare office in an industrial-type building. (There are no crystal balls, veils, or other esoteric apparatus!) May I describe his approach as very down-to-earth, even when he appears to be in direct contact with 'the other side'?

He also tells me that I will write a book detailing my experience with this cancer. This stuns me as I have never written anything other than term papers and business reports. But he is adamant and says many people will be helped by me sharing my journey.

I really have trouble believing this one, but try to keep an open mind to see where it goes!

(By the way, he also foretells several other personal things that happen exactly as he predicted within a few months' time, so I am able to put great faith in all he told me.)

CHEMO
RECOMMENDED

I continue to see the oncologist every four months with the occasional CT scan thrown in and my condition stays excellent.

At one point, my doctor, being the professional he is, tells me he has presented my case to the hospital tumour board (composed of his colleagues), and they recommend that I begin chemotherapy.

I understand their reasoning to be based on the seriousness of this disease and my atypical evolution. As I was told in the beginning, this lymphoma normally requires treatment immediately upon diagnosis. Most people arrive with clear indications of disease, such as sudden weight loss. However, since I am feeling perfectly well, have not lost one ounce and no one can assure me of the value of starting treatment now, I refuse. The doctors and all of the medical literature clearly state that this particular type of chemo does not cure, it buys time. The idea of making myself feel very ill because of non-essential chemo, when I have already been told this lymphoma is incurable, does not add up for me. My oncologist does not press the issue and I am grateful for his understanding.

ALTERNATIVES
FROM OUTSIDE THE BOX

During this time, I also consult other types of therapists. My gut feeling of whether I feel they might help guides me, but the fact that they cannot harm is the number one criterion.

I see a lovely Chinese acupuncturist several times and feel increased energy.

I continue to see my marvellous osteopath, Frédéric, who personifies sensitivity and healing. He helps with an ongoing back problem and applies pressure on the enlarged ganglions to prevent them from adhering. Another osteopath who works solely on the energy level and is very connected spiritually helps in an entirely different manner. I often put myself in my hypnotic state when I'm with her, and I experience feelings of healing and well-being that are hard to express.

CLAUDIA RAINVILLE

And of course, during this time, I am reading four books by Claudia Rainville, as recommended by Bernard. Fortunately, her work is readily available in Montreal in French.

Her Great Dictionary of Meta-Medecine *(Grand dictionnaire de la Métamédecine)* is a guide that points you towards an understanding of the emotional issues underlying each disease or body part affected.

Once you have looked up the specific illness or body part which concerns you, she offers an explanation and questions to ask yourself. She clearly describes what she believes to be the emotional causes of each illness in detail.

This fits in with what I had already intuitively sensed myself, and with what Bernard had described to me.

One of her explanations for lymphoma resonates particularly strongly with me. It concerns feelings of abandonment and not having felt protected.

In all of my significant personal relationships, whenever there has been a serious problem or separation, I have always felt a huge sense of abandonment, often quite out of proportion to the circumstances.

As Claudia explains, the role of the lymph system is to protect and defend the body. Therefore, my lymphoma arises from my emotional feeling of being unprotected.

Her book asks certain questions about feelings of not being protected to allow you to try and identify a related causal childhood experience.

I understand her approach to say that a very strong emotional reaction in adulthood will resonate with, and be caused by, the original emotional reaction in childhood, usually early childhood.

As I had a very happy childhood, the only thing that sticks in my thoughts is the difficulty in my relationship with my Dad.

For some reason, there was always some tension between us even though we cared deeply for one another. I was certainly loved and cherished as the youngest of four children with only five years between us all. My relationship with my Mom was fantastic, we were on the same wavelength and shared great complicity.

These questions are now simmering in the back of my mind concerning feeling unprotected and abandoned in my early years.

AN IMPROBABLE
BREAKTHROUGH

One major difficulty I am having revolves around my memory. I have *very* few memories of my childhood and consequently cannot summon up childhood experiences to explain why I have felt abandoned when relationships stumbled.

My favourite place is my cottage (or camp, as we refer to it) at Silver Islet, about one hundred kilometers from Thunder Bay in Northwestern Ontario.

I have been there every summer of my life and either am related to, or have known for many years, almost everyone there. I face the grandeur of Lake Superior in peaceful surroundings.

One day during my summer vacation there, I lie fully relaxed in a self-hypnotic state and let thoughts roam freely in my head.

Suddenly I remember one of the tales often recounted amidst great laughter when my family got together.

It is a childhood scene where I was around two or three years old.

As children we spent most of the day running free.

When I was little, I did not want to take precious time while playing outside to return to the house to pee, and so just did like the boys and pulled down my panties and peed outside.

Apparently, this was totally unacceptable behaviour for a small girl and I was reprimanded many times.

To "cure" me of this bad habit, one day my Dad (the "protector" figure supreme for a child) pretended to telephone the hospital in front of the whole family to ask them to take me back as I did not obey. (Of course, we all believed that babies came from the hospital—sex education was stilted to non-existent then). As the story goes, everyone was crying and my older siblings were begging him not to send me away. The threat was obviously effective as it was never repeated.

I do not actually remember this myself as it must have been so terrifying for me. I have completely sublimated the memory. And even though this story was told and re-told at family gatherings, no-one, least of all me, seemed to think anything about how traumatic this would seem to a small child!

Well how is that for discovering why I feel abandoned and unprotected during times of emotional stress? As I said before, my parents loved us and did absolutely everything they could for us. My Dad was a very effective problem solver and he took care of this situation efficiently. No one could have predicted the effect it had on me many years later. But even though I cannot remember this happening, it was clearly significant in the ongoing relationship I had with my Dad.

So, now I have an understanding of what is behind my over-reaction to this failed relationship that triggered my cancer. The question is, "what do I do now?"

THERAPEUTIC RE-ENACTMENT

Claudia Rainville wrote another book that describes her therapeutic approach to heal the original emotional reaction. It is entitled *Métamédecine. Les outils thérapeutiques* or Meta-Medicine, Therapeutic Tools.

I immediately dive in and try to heal myself by using this method. I find it fascinating, although somewhat difficult to do on my own. But I still make a lot of progress and feel a definite lessening of tension.

In early January 2013, however, I suddenly awake one morning knowing I must meet Claudia and pursue my healing with her.

Through the wonders of the Internet, I find someone who works with her in France and ask her to forward my request to Claudia. By day's end, Claudia and I are corresponding and over the next few weeks, I make arrangements to go and see her in the Dominican Republic. Claudia spends several winter months there to devote to her writing, but she agrees to see me during that time.

What a bonus! Escaping the Canadian winter for a week and hopefully deepening my understanding of her approach?

Claudia is very open and welcoming when I meet her, and we hit it off immediately. We have one therapeutic session together which closely follows the model I had used from her book.

The emotional impact of this session is however much stronger, with Claudia taking the role of my father during the event of him calling the hospital to ask them to take me back. Afterwards she clarifies with me what beliefs I have developed as a result of his action.

I finally feel I have explored in depth how to move forward and change my behaviour regarding relationships and gained a clear understanding of it. Of course, it still remains a tough thing to actually *do*, but awareness is the first and vital step.

Claudia also unearths for me a belief I had unconsciously developed because of this emotional trauma with my Dad, which was that "I cannot win."

I now recognize this pattern throughout my life, with my Dad as well as with other authority figures— especially men.

It is also essential for me to change this belief with regards to the lymphoma. I must understand deep within that I can and will "win" in this situation. And I have the enormous advantage of having Bernard in my life with his accurate and immensely reassuring predictions.

THE ROLLER COASTER

Of course, I come away from my time with Claudia fully expecting my lumps to disappear overnight. Did I mention that I am an optimist? That does not happen, but life goes on and I am happy continuing to work, enjoying my friends, and thinking long and hard about all I am learning.

At the same time, the hope/fear roller-coaster affects me directly. It is rare for me to stay "up" for more than a week at a time. It seems we hear of a new cancer diagnosis every day, followed by stories of wonderful people suffering and dying.

The prevalence of this disease makes it sound like our century's plague.

I have never again plumbed the depths of terror I lived in for the first two years after diagnosis. But my confidence in my healing ebbs and flows. When I am in my good space, it is really the most wonderful sort of high. I am so grateful for my life, family, friends, appetite—you name it, I am grateful for it!

But it is a bit alarming how a very small thing can quickly bring me down to a fretting, worry-filled level. This is an ongoing challenge and it is actually quite fun to discover how to avoid/circumvent/ignore the negative messages.

I avidly read my horoscope in the two newspapers I receive every day, and select the one I prefer as being accurate. Any article concerning "spontaneous remissions," I read fully and adapt to my circumstances.

People who are in any way negative, depressing or not supportive of my path are either excluded from being privy to my thoughts or avoided altogether. When that is not possible, I quickly imagine myself cloaked in a protective white light that does not allow their negativity to attain me. I may have gotten the idea from Harry Potter—just goes to show that whatever works for you is good!

But seriously, my mainstay is to go back to my self-hypnosis, give myself positive messages and listen carefully to my intuition. It is rare that I cannot transform my fears back to hope when I do this. At last night's yoga session, during *shavasana* (my best position), my intuition suddenly told me that I simply have to *believe* that I will be healed. It is an article of faith and cannot be explained or rationalized. It is a belief, the same as a religious one.

So, here is my new way to live, without doubt. This morning, it feels right. I am not "tempting the gods," I am simply living my strong belief.

TRADITIONAL VS ALTERNATIVE

I also continue seeing the oncologist regularly.

It seems to me that our approach to sickness looks a lot like the old Indian fable of the blind men and the elephant. Remember how each one perceived and defined the animal according to which part of the body he touched. The one who touched the leg thought it must be like a tree; the one who touched the trunk said it had to be like a snake, and so on.

When you are the patient in our Western medical system it can feel much like that. Increased specialization sends you to a host of different experts who seem to know a great deal about the small body part or disease they have studied. I guess theoretically the family doctor is supposed to be the one person who sees you as a whole being, but in fact, when you get a serious illness, you are somewhat thrown to the wolves

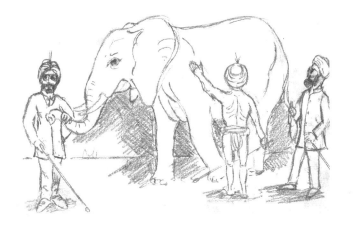

of the many different specialists and left quite on your own to try to figure things out.

My family doctor does not accompany me to those appointments nor tell me what questions to ask, nor what to keep track of. It can be bewildering, and one must be in good enough health to navigate this system. Having your own personal advocate accompany you, coupled with extensive note-taking, is a huge asset.

Some alternative or holistic treatment practitioners seem to try to look at your entire being, but too often, each one wants you to commit exclusively to their proposed regimen. And I am always wary of those who insist their way is the only way.

One of the reasons I so appreciate my osteopath, Frédéric, is because he has such in-depth knowledge of the whole body, and he incorporates traditional medicine as appropriate. Some alternatives can become too doctrinal and not take advantage of the help that can be provided by other options or by classic Western medicine.

Again, my first criterion to trying something is to ensure it will not cause me harm. But once that is taken care of, an open and even adventurous spirit can lead to many positive surprises.

My sessions with Nicole, my non-conventional osteopath, have helped me tremendously. She is a deeply spiritual, intuitive woman who has a healing touch.

Our many conversations about my current states of emotion always contribute to greater understanding and progress on my journey to well-being. While being treated by her and in my state of self-hypnosis, I have several amazing experiences. Whether I call it intuition or being in touch with the universal energy, I gain deep insights.

One time during treatment, she suddenly asks me what I am feeling. Out of the clear blue with no forethought, I reply that I feel a pressure around my solar plexus. A few seconds later, I feel this pressure go to the right side of my heart and know I am being healed. When she asks me what I am being cured of, I immediately respond that it is my relationship with my father. I had no idea I was even thinking of him, but I *know* this is my truth. I cannot explain how or why I know this, but it is an absolute given for me.

THE ONCOLOGIST
RAISES A QUESTION

In December 2013, I see my oncologist for a six-month follow-up. He feels the ganglions have grown a bit and says it is likely time to begin treatment. He schedules a CT scan and a subsequent appointment in late January in order to confirm his opinion.

Meanwhile, I acknowledge to myself that I am having more symptoms and discomfort.

I surprise myself by seeming to accept the possible need for treatment with a measure of equanimity, given my sheer refusal and terror of chemotherapy up to now. I believe it is because of my conversations with Bernard. So I immediately make plans to discuss all of this with him.

CHOP OR NOT

We talk by Skype in early January 2014.

As usual, Bernard "sees" clearly what will take place, and predicts that I will be starting chemo, but not for several weeks. He is quite precise in fact, saying I will begin in April and finish either in July or August. Also, he indicates that I will not be unduly affected by this chemo and will not find it too difficult. He also reassures me that I will be able to find a new type of treatment here in Montreal other than the old CHOP regimen—a matter of huge importance to me. (Each letter of CHOP refers to a chemotherapy drug).

After talking with Bernard, I charge forward to more fully investigate the newer types of chemo and how I will be able to access them. I am adamant about not undergoing the CHOP chemo. This was first an intuitive, gut reaction. But also a good friend had

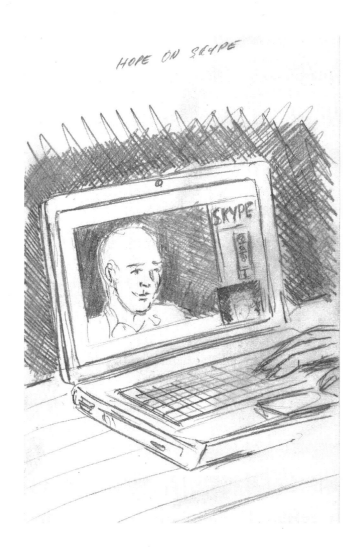

recently developed terminal leukemia after the CHOP treatment for his lymphoma.

Hours turn into days spent poring over Internet sites and learning a whole new vocabulary. Who in the world could ever dream up these names for drugs? Apparently they are meaningful to those who spend their lives in this field, but I can vouch that they do not exactly roll off your tongue. What's more these unpronounceable drugs end up with two names, one being for commercial purposes.

I discover the newer drug Bendamustine, which was developed in East Germany during the Cold War years and has been used there for quite a while. It is based on the mustard gas used to kill soldiers in the war. Now that does not sound very enticing, but the results are actually quite impressive. It was not known in Western medicine until the reunification of Germany. Being a newer drug in Canada, Bendamustine is much more costly than CHOP, and for that reason it is not currently given in Quebec for first-time treatment.

After finding out the name of the pharmaceutical company distributing this drug in Montreal, I speak with a representative about how to get access to it. He is very kind, but offers no options. The drug is only sold to the proper government agencies, not to an individual. By the end of the call, I am weeping in frustration.

I telephone the doctor I had seen in Boston two years earlier and he tells me they are using Bendamustine frequently for this type of situation.

So now I know at least that I have the possibility of going to Boston for treatment (at *huge* cost, both financial and because it would mean being away from my own home). Later my oncologist informs me that I could buy this drug from my own hospital, but would need to go to a private clinic to have it administered.

THE TREATMENT
IN THE HAYSTACK

After many, many hours spent searching on the Internet, I discover a pharmaceutical research protocol for using the drug Bendamustine with Rituximab, plus a very new drug under investigation (Ibrutinib).

It takes many more hours to find out the name of the hematologist/oncologist responsible for this study in Montreal and then to determine if I am eligible.

This study calls for newly-diagnosed Mantle Cell Lymphoma patients who have had no prior treatment. Since I was diagnosed four years earlier, I would probably fall through the cracks and not be considered.

I presume that this particular eligibility criterion stemmed from the fact that, typically, newly-diagnosed patients require treatment immediately. However, since I have had no treatment to date, I feel I should be included as a potential candidate.

Because all of this takes such a great deal of time, and I continually worry that those nasty little cancer cells must be replicating madly, I am now in a state of high anxiety.

I nearly rip the head off of the oncologist responsible for this study when he finally calls to say I can see him but not before several weeks. It has now been over ten weeks that I know I need to begin chemo and I have spent full days attempting to understand and access the best type. In fact, I tell him to forget it because the whole procedure is taking too long.

OOPS!

Of course, once I calm down later that evening, I realize I must apologize. So I send him an e-mail explaining the reasons for my behaviour and asking for his forbearance. Luckily, he does not hold a grudge and tells me an appointment will be scheduled.

Even though chemotherapy will begin within the next several weeks, I do not feel anxiety about it. At the most, a foreboding of some unpleasant days ahead because of the treatment, but almost a relief that I will get this underway, and afterwards be healed. Of course, my talks with Bernard are the major contributor to this equanimity.

ONCOLOGIST NUMBER THREE

When I first meet my new oncologist at a different hospital, he explains the research protocol in detail. He seems like a good guy and that helps because I really liked my second oncologist. I think doctors underestimate the value placed by a patient on their relationship.

The possible side effects fill pages and pages, with all of them going from bad to worse, ending with death. However, as he points out, if you read the same such list for an aspirin, it would not seem much better.

The good news is that I have access to the drug Bendamustine, and all is paid for by the pharmaceutical company and administered directly in the hospital. There are ongoing follow-ups, blood tests, and scans on a regular basis (read *too* often).

Sadly, the bad news is there will be more bone marrow biopsies. That is certainly a reason to hesitate.

After the obligatory 24-hour reflection period, I return the following day to actually sign the document, and the protocol is officially set in motion.

Too late to turn back? Not really, but now I just want to get this over with.

GERMS AND TESTS

Before anything can actually start, I must attend a general information meeting on chemotherapy at the hospital. This explains how to protect oneself from the risk of infection, because our immune system is significantly weakened during chemo. It also provides me with the unexpected opportunity to meet another patient who is part of the same research protocol. This is fun because otherwise, we are never told who else is on the same study. I believe this is part of the protocol in order to avoid us influencing, or being influenced by, another patient. He and his wife seem like good people and we share our stories of life in the cancer lane at this early stage.

A nutritionist runs through some issues on eating well during chemo and then we get to the juicy part.

Wow, the information about nasty germs lurking everywhere is extensive.

Acting like a combination of Howard Hughes and Niles, the obsessive/compulsive brother from the TV sitcom Frasier, should have me covered in this category!

Who knew you had to scrub all lids of cans with soap and hot water before opening? You would not believe just how disgustingly filthy they are.

I learn to approach my friends with my hands held up to ward off any attempts at hugging. In Quebec, we are very kissy-face, and a kiss on each cheek is the standard greeting. No more of that!

Poisonous doorknobs and elevator buttons must be neutralized.

What not to eat? Good-bye sushi, delicious unpasteurized cheese, and honey. Out with the rare meat!

Gloves and masks enter my life for the next months. I cannot even garden without them.

Another CT scan must be taken, as it is a requirement of the protocol that it be done within a very short time-frame before beginning treatment.

I find this upsetting as I had just had a scan two months earlier and hate the thought of all that radiation. But there is no choice allowed, the research protocol is king. As I am discovering, participating in this type of study definitely has its up-sides and downs-sides.

Despite my several CT scans taken at my previous hospital, this time I develop an allergic reaction. I turn beet-red and my face and torso are very itchy, but the up-side is my face is so swollen: I have not one single wrinkle! I race to the pharmacy and load up on Benadryl. For future scans, I will require a mix of CT and MRI, in order to avoid the iodine contrast that caused my allergic reaction.

For the bone marrow biopsy, I ask Corinne, an accomplished yoga teacher and friend, to accompany me to help me do yoga breathing during the torture.

This turns out to be highly ineffective, as the doc kicks her out of the tiny room beforehand so as to ensure sterile conditions.

I still try the breathing on my own, but it is somewhat ragged. At least this time, the doctor has given me an injection to help reduce the pain. All I can say about the painkiller is that it is much better than not having one.

All has been completed, and finally I am ready to begin treatment.

The ordeal of waiting to start treatment probably appears perfectly ordinary to those who organize such things. It is another story for the one waiting, feeling those horrid little cells multiplying day and night. Surely something can be done to improve this wait time and thereby reduce the anxiety build-up.

FASTING AND CHEMO

Meanwhile, I have discovered some research being done involving fasting before and during chemo.

Two years ago, during a visit to Paris with Anik, I had actually noticed, by chance, a very small article on fasting during chemotherapy.

This research from the University of Southern California has come out of the field of geriatrics, and it demonstrated that lab rats that are very thin have a longer life span than those of normal weight.

With regards to chemotherapy, the theory is that after fasting for at least forty-eight hours, normal healthy cells in our body, fearing starvation, go into survival mode whereby they can form a sort of safety barrier around themselves. This barrier also diminishes the side effects of the chemo. Since the cancerous cells, also vulnerable due to the fasting, are unable to go into this protective mode and they respond even more strongly to the chemo. Obviously, more effective chemo combined with lessened side effects sounds good to me.

Many Internet hours later, I contact those responsible at the Mayo Clinic to discuss the rationale and criteria for inclusion in their upcoming study on this issue. The very fact that I will be swallowing four pills each day of the drug under investigation as part of my treatment (which may be chemo or a placebo) naturally makes me ineligible. It goes without saying that I cannot fast every day for twenty-four weeks!

The theory and rationale nonetheless appeal strongly to me, so I decide to fast before and during the six periods of intravenous chemo (Bendamustine and Rituximab). In my case, this requires fasting (no food, only *lots* of water) from Saturday evening to Thursday suppertime every twenty-eight days for six cycles.

Imagine how this will help my waistline, if nothing else.

I read a few books and online articles to have an idea what to expect and am given some tips by my yoga instructor.

Fasting is hardly a new idea. It has been a component of most religions for centuries—think of Lent for Christians and Ramadan for Muslims. It is widely accepted as a health measure today, especially in Germany and Russia. Many, many people fast regularly, for widely varying time frames, even though it is only now becoming more accepted in North America.

I learn that generally hunger is not felt after two days and that there are usually side effects such as headache, nausea, and dizziness during the first two to three days.

I thoroughly enjoy my dinner on the Saturday night before the upcoming IV chemo on Tuesday, and then only drink water, lots of water.

One odd thing I notice is just how much free time I suddenly have. We don't realize how much time is taken up with food planning, shopping, preparation, and clean-up. Fasting should really be called slowing.

As predicted, my hunger pangs only last for about thirty hours, and I do feel light-headed much of the time.

CHEMO

I arrive for my first day of intravenous chemotherapy accompanied by my wonderful friend Sylvie, and have only ingested water for the past fifty-six hours. The good news is I feel so dizzy and nauseated from the fasting that I cannot worry about the chemo. The bad news (especially for Sylvie) is that I throw up before the chemo even begins. Once that is over, however, I feel much better (frankly, there was not much other than water to evacuate!) and head in to finally get this process underway.

I hit pay dirt by having the most fabulous nurse for my first time, Trish. She inspires confidence, explains each step of the way, and gets the IV inserted without problem. This reassures me as my doctor was worried I might need a catheter (Picc line) because my veins are fairly small. Trish also has a wonderful sense of humour, and with her sidekick, Michelle, I am extremely well cared for.

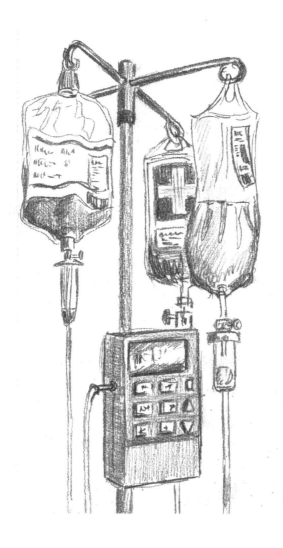

To my consternation, I am given three Tylenol, thirty minutes of IV Benadryl, followed by another thirty minutes of IV hydrocortisone before we even get to the chemo. All this is to prevent a possible allergic reaction.

I hate taking pills and doubt I have ever swallowed three Tylenol at the same time in my entire life. When I protest gingerly, I am politely reminded that the protocol is not to be questioned, only strictly followed.

Finally, Trish gets into her Hazmat type of suit and hooks up the first chemo drug-Rituximab. It is administered very slowly because of the worry of an allergic reaction. I'm not sure what to expect, but I feel nothing untoward.

Around three hours later, I am given two potent anti-nausea pills and shortly thereafter, the other drug, Bendamustine, is hooked up. This drug can be given quickly, so one hour later, I can finally be "un-hooked" and am more than ready to head home. I feel full and uncomfortable. Exhaustion has set in. The hospital pharmacy has supplied me with another sort of anti-nausea pill to take at home, and a few hours later, I definitely need it.

That night, I have terrific pain in my legs and hips, something I was not really expecting and that no one had warned me about. Sleep is out of the question.

The next morning, back we go for the second day of treatment, only Bendamustine, preceded of course by the potent anti-nausea pills.

Thankfully this day is shorter and I can come home to literally collapse in bed for a few hours.

The atmosphere in the treatment room is surprisingly upbeat. We patients often chat among ourselves and the nurses are very friendly and efficient. Every now and then, someone has a hard time and that is respected by all.

I see every imaginable type of wig, hat, bald head, and artfully arranged scarf. For women, losing our hair can be tough psychologically. It adds another layer of stress to our anxiety. As one of the lucky ones, I will not lose my hair with this type of chemo and this provides an appreciated boost.

To make it worse, my scarf skills are somewhat disastrous—I simply have no ability in cleverly knotting scarves. Scarf-tying has always been a long-standing family joke, starting with my Mom.

Every day, I swallow four pills around the same time in the morning, not sure if it is the chemo study drug (Ibrutinib) or a placebo.

The drug trial calls for the intravenous drugs to be given every twenty-eight days for six cycles, followed

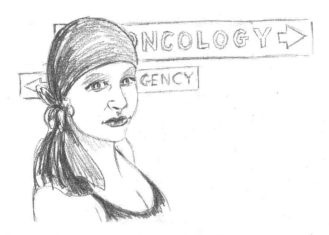

by a maintenance regimen of the IV Rituximab for two years, given every eight weeks. Also, the daily placebo/Ibrutinib continues until the end of the study or, I believe, 'till death do us part! I plan for that to be a long time off.

The two days of actual treatment are fairly tough. I feel so filled with chemicals, even before the chemo starts.

I attempt to put my head into a calm state whereby I do not think about what is happening, just sort of drift along. At the same time, I am fully aware of everything and closely monitor what drug is given when. The nausea is manageable with the pills, but I always feel full and loggy.

Too many people are so sick before they even begin treatment. Many have financial or personal worries on top of their health problems. Those who do not have a strong support group of family and friends are tremendously disadvantaged. I would never dare complain about my situation when I see what others are going through. I cannot even imagine how someone like a single mom with limited means can get through this. I am truly grateful for my much easier time and all of the help and support I receive.

BECOMING HUMAN AGAIN

On the Thursday at dinnertime, I can eat once again. I do not feel hunger, but look forward to tasting something delicious and sharing a mealtime with others.

About three or four days after treatment, I start to feel closer to being human again, with the main side-effect being extreme tiredness. Daily naps have come to mean a deep sleep of at least two hours, followed by a night of ten hours.

The following Monday, I decide to go to my Pilates class, a bit unsure of what I will be able to accomplish, but wanting to exercise if possible and still feel some sense of normality in my life.

I am able to function at about fifty percent of my usual ability, and feel exhausted but exhilarated. The main drawback is dizziness when I change position.

Two weeks later, I begin an eight-week course on mindful meditation. It proves to be an interesting adjunct to my self-hypnosis, with the emphasis on living in the present moment and discarding all judgement of others.

I am so living the present moment right now!

Judgement of others is a work in progress especially with one particular hospital employee whose work ethic is very different from mine.

Over the next three weeks, I can feel myself slowly climbing back up, and then, of course, just as I am feeling fairly well, we begin again.

The most exciting news however is that the ganglions have visibly shrunk. My doctor says that is typical of Bendamustine and posits that the severe pain in my legs and hips after that first treatment was the drug working in the bone marrow. If so, I will not complain about that again.

On the third cycle, after fasting for the first three days, I am feeling so dizzy and nauseated that I decide to stop the fasting. Coupled with chemotherapy, it is not an easy thing to go through and as soon as I drink a glass of orange juice, I am a changed person. No more nausea or dizziness. No doubt it is very radical for my body to suddenly try to adjust to such lengthy periods without nourishment so closely repeated.

So that is the end of the fasting for me for now. But I am really proud to have accomplished it for these two and a half times. I may never know for sure the extent to which it has helped me, but my intuition tells me it was the right thing to do.

After treatment number four, it is July. My sister Anne is having a serious birthday at our summer place, Silver Islet. A serious birthday means that it ends with a zero.

My doctor advises I may attend if I feel up to it. I am already sad at not spending my summer there as usual, and Anne's birthday is important to me, so I decide to give it a go. Armed with masks, gloves, a more expensive seat at the very front of the plane, (hopefully far from those pesky germs), I take off for the cottage.

All goes well and I truly believe that my eight days there accomplish a great deal for me health-wise. In any case it helps immensely morale-wise, and how can that not improve my physical well-being?

Only two more sessions to go! For some odd reason, the fifth treatment is tougher than I expected. Not sure if that is because of a build-up of the chemicals or just a certain weariness on my part.

Finally, the last of the "big" treatments arrives at the very end of August, exactly on schedule with what

Bernard predicted last January before I was even told by my doctor that I definitely required chemotherapy.

I can hardly believe it and yet the positive build-up I expect does not happen. One reason is the very long wait before I actually get into the treatment room.

Chemotherapy tradition calls for a person to ring a bell at the end of the last treatment. I do not ring the bell upon leaving as I am too tired and most of the others have already gone home. What's more, I will be back in eight weeks. I cannot even feel elated a couple of days later.

SIX CYCLES BEHIND ME

It only hits me about two weeks after it is over that this major part of the ordeal is behind me. I don't really feel a huge sense of relief because there are the tests to "look forward" to.

If the CT/MRI scan is good, they will request a PET scan—positron emission tomography for insiders. Otherwise, they keep waiting to see if you will show any further improvement.

When I receive the CT/MRI scan results, I am very disheartened by the wording which sounds to me like it does not specify excellent results. Furthermore, since the results were not forwarded to my doctor when they should have been, I am forced to wait another hour on top of the two already gone by. Then, he gives me the results while standing in a very busy, noisy hallway, since by then our room is being used by others. He says the results are positive, but the report does not sound that positive to me. Is my reaction caused by a build-up of anxiety, compounded by the lengthy wait?

I send him an e-mail a couple of days later asking whether he could clarify the radiology report with the fellow who wrote it, but do not hear back from him. My attempt to question the radiologist directly on this falls flat, as medical protocol trumps communication directly with the patient. However perhaps it has a good effect as I am scheduled for a PET scan within a few weeks.

CHAMPAGNE

Meanwhile, I have planned a Skype call with my ever-prescient Bernard.

He immediately tells me that although I must finish the two years of maintenance IV chemo, the cancer will be in total remission. I am not to worry about it further.

And so I go into the PET scan with peace of mind. Sure enough, at my follow-up appointment with the oncologist in late October, he tells me the PET-scan results are excellent and I am in remission. Of course, I simply know I am cured, but understandably, that word cannot pass his lips.

I feel lighter than air and am floating. Upon arriving home, I announce the great news to people who work in my building, and to a complete stranger in the elevator! He graciously congratulates me.

The one-day maintenance chemo every eight weeks is not really taxing. The day itself is wearisome, but already the following day, I am feeling much better.

My December treatment is preceded by the dreaded bone marrow biopsy—the final one. Sadly, it does not become easier over time, and I decide to not muffle my screams.

Afterwards, I announce to my doc that I will never have another one. Now apparently that really is "tempting the gods" because when I return the next day for the actual treatment, I learn that there was a mistake the previous day. Yes, the biopsy must be re-done in part! At least it is not quite as painful as having the complete one.

The only up-side—but it is highly significant—comes when my doc says the results from the previous day show NO cancer cells in my bone marrow.

My e-mail account just might have overheated today, what with my message to everyone and their joyful replies.

Over the next days, champagne and gratitude are shared with my wide group of friends and for the moment, only gratitude with my far-flung family. That will change with our Christmas holidays together. There is nothing like champagne to celebrate being alive and well!

BACK TO BERNARD
(THE MEDIUM)

Bernard also tells me to get busy with my book, in no uncertain terms. Did I mention he can be somewhat pushy when he feels I am not listening to him? He assures me that my story will be helpful to others who are facing health challenges. I have written a few tentative pages, feeling very unsure of myself, but as Bernard has not been off the mark about one single thing over the last years, I carry on as best I can.

The most difficult thing for me is to put into words exactly what my beliefs are. I am quite clear on what I do *not* believe, but find it difficult to express what I really do believe. When I mention this to Bernard, he recommends I find a book by Wayne Dyer called *The Power of Intention*.

I dive in. His work is enlightening. He underscores the immense importance of our thoughts, and the devastating effects of negative thoughts.

His idea of what constitutes intention is completely different from what we normally think of, namely a strong will power or a significant determination. As he says, "Imagine that intention is not something you do, but rather a force that exists in the Universe as an invisible field of energy." It sounds to me like the pattern or source behind all of life.

For several years now, I have been edging my way towards the idea that our thoughts are of supreme importance, but this really brings it home.

FAMILY AND FRIENDS

My sister Anne has been my stalwart and the very model of loving support.

My sister Mary has exemplified courage and determination in dealing with multiple sclerosis over the past fifty years.

The rest of my far-flung family has called, prayed, e-mailed, and offered to come and help in any and every way.

My out-of-town friends were willing to put their lives on hold and come to accompany me to the chemo sessions.

My amazing friends here at home have fed me, consoled me, sat with me through long, boring chemo sessions, made me laugh, let me cry, and carefully hugged me.

I have been nourished by them all, in every sense of the word.

I have gone through these past ten years living alone. This was a worry for some of my family and friends. Yes, a broad shoulder to cry on and strong arms to wrap around me would have been a bonus at many moments. But I could not have asked for more than what they gave me.

And yet, I was given more. I was given the chance to understand how to better live my life. This is the surprising bonus of disease!

I believe we are meant to grow and learn and expand during our lifetime.

I joke that I do not wish to "fail" the test, live unhappily, and come back in my next life forced to repeat the same lessons! Every single moment we experience is an opportunity to question and grow.

No, I do not understand the horrible suffering endured by so many people. Karma is interesting and offers an explanation, but not one I feel I comprehend adequately.

The goal is to understand and feel we are truly all connected at the level of universal energy. At this level, we can only experience love for each and all, and therefore judgement of the other is not possible.

How I wish I could live this way more often. It is easy when I am in self-hypnosis, and it is slowly developing more and more in my daily life.

I have the great good fortune to have a couple of friends in my life who unwittingly model such behaviour for me. I take advantage of every lesson (which, even better, almost always involves lunch or dinner). After my experience of fasting, combined with my innate love of good food, I try to combine every lesson with an interesting menu.

THE NEED TO UNDERSTAND

Psychology and human behaviour books have interested me for a very long time. There are periods of bulimia when I positively gorge myself, and other times when I take a break. This need to understand human behaviour as much as possible has been part of me since university and has never diminished.

I have read many books, and of course, have made myself a major subject of study, as I could ask myself those difficult or indiscreet questions and develop theories to be investigated. Along the way, I have always had the great luck to find a very few other kindred spirits who share my enthusiasm. My cousin, Cath, has been a helpful catalyst over these many years of reading and sharing theories. We bounce ideas off each other freely with no criticism ever.

My deep need to understand may help explain my original search to comprehend what is behind my illness.

Several of the books suggested to me over the past five years have resonated particularly strongly with me, especially those of Dr. David Hawkins. Each of us needs to explore different readings to discover just what works for us.

HOPE

Let me talk to you about hope.

I get upset and angry when I hear the expression "false" hope. This very idea is ridiculous to me because hope is an expectation and cannot be "false."

Hope is a belief and like all beliefs, by definition is not proven. When something is proven, it is no longer a belief.

We all know of someone whose hope seemed to carry them through a seemingly impossible situation. Should an undesirable outcome occur, this does not mean that the hope was false or that it was not helpful. How much better to live with the uplifting, and I believe, physically beneficial effects of hope for the longest possible time.

To live without hope is to live in despair. Why would anyone want that for themselves or others? This does not mean that one cannot be accepting of death.

For me, and I suspect for many people, suffering is the great difficulty, death is not the worst thing to face.

In early 2010, after I was diagnosed with Mantle Cell Lymphoma, I was told it is incurable and that my life expectancy was six years. This unasked-for news propelled me into a state of high anxiety and despondency.

It is most bizarre and unsettling to suddenly be given your best-before date, especially when you feel perfectly well. Add to that the idea of having six years—not six months—and you do not know what to do with this amount of time. When I was fearful, anxious or sad, I felt terrible to be wasting precious time. I was certain that the six years in question would be filled with horrible treatments that would prevent me from benefiting from those years.

As it turns out, I did not have any form of treatment or discomfort until four years later.

Even if I had asked for the estimate of my life expectancy, why would my doctor not tell me the numbers while explaining that six years is a very long time in medicine, and that new discoveries for treating cancer are being made every day? The type of chemo given to me in 2014 was not known here in 2010. And what about today? Can anyone possibly think I should have lived those years without hope?

I believe that any medical doctor worthy of the title will not judge a situation as without hope until the end of life is very obvious and within a few short weeks. The impact of a doctor telling you that there is no hope, or not to try alternative options because they hold out "false" hope, is devastating and arrogant on the doctor's part.

Family members and friends will also have a major negative effect if they ridicule or otherwise do not support the hopes of a patient. Sometimes a seriously ill person will be despairing and any hope provided by others can have unexpected and fruitful results.

There have always existed "miraculous" situations, by which I mean cures that are inexplicable to us with the scientific knowledge of today.

Some of the alternative types of help I have used over the past years would be considered frivolous or even ridiculous by some. As I have said, my first criterion has always been to ensure that what I was trying could not harm me physically or emotionally.

I also ensured that whatever I tried was not onerous financially or provided at an exaggerated cost. For example, one person who was highly recommended to me did not pass muster as her foremost concern was with money.

Having said that, I was immensely helped by actually doing something, taking some sort of action.

When I first began meeting with the eccentric "Professeur Tournesol" in France, he gave me hope. I will never know for sure how my health has actually benefited from his interventions; however, my outlook on life improved immensely. And I am positive that this helps in terms of physical as well as mental health.

To live without hope is not sustainable. Following all of my conversations with Bernard, I had greatly renewed energy and happiness, not least because of the hopeful situations he described.

LAUGHTER

Laughter is essential to life as I know it. A day without a really good laugh is not fulfilling, not to mention *dull*!

So many common events that seem deathly serious to us appear totally different when we step back and look at the situation as an observer. Very often, the seriousness turns straight to chuckles as we wonder why we got so upset about what really is fairly trivial in the grand scheme of things.

One piece of advice I regularly use is to say, "Will I care about or even remember this in five years' time?" And since my memory is not reliable, I usually already know the answer!

Bringing humour to a situation allows us to gain perspective and distance from it. This also applies to what life and death moments really are.

Using laughter whenever possible helps us both physically and mentally. During chemo treatments, this was one of the things I most appreciated, the banter and chuckles between the nurses and patients and among the patients. All of us who were not too ill during treatment truly enjoyed sharing these moments.

I try to see the funny side of any given situation, and I also try to look for situations which will give me a laugh. Violent movies, books or news are *verboten*, funny films are actively sought. When I think about my friends—as extremely diverse as they are—one common thread is a great sense of humour.

The books by Dr. Norman Cousins, published many years ago, bear witness to the importance of humour in health.

Even when events in our lives have seemed to conspire against us, black humour is better than none!

POSITIVE THOUGHTS

I believe that both hope and humour fill our body with tremendously positive thoughts that directly impact our physical and mental well-being. The impact of negativity, violence, unkindness, guilt or remorse, for example, cannot be over-estimated in their huge effect on our health.

We are *not* separate from our thoughts and emotions in the physical sense. They are just as much a part of us as our arms and legs. The energy of our thoughts has been measurably demonstrated many times over.

Double-blind studies of Buddhist monks in the U.S. have shown impressive results.

The effect of stress on our bodies is well documented. Stress does not exist in reality, so what causes it? Our own thoughts and emotions. Even in a very difficult situation, each individual may have a widely different reaction, each reaction brought about by our own thoughts and feelings. If we can recognize this and channel our thoughts and emotions to a higher level, the physical effects will be diminished or even negated.

A FIGHT? I BEG TO DISAGREE

When we hear our diagnosis of cancer, along with the fear, our first thoughts are to mount an attack.

How many times do we read of a person who so courageously "fought" their cancer?

While I have the utmost respect and personal understanding of the anxiety, pain and discomfort involved, coupled with the courage to hope to recover, I think there is definitely an element out of line with this approach.

Instead of seeing our illness as a dreaded foe requiring all our energy to fight, we can consider it as an event that can teach us.

I believe we must look inward at our emotional states and thought patterns, both current and past to discover just how they have affected us health-wise.

Our "fight" should be with ourselves if you will, rather than against the illness.

The illness is an opportunity to delve inside emotionally and seek understanding of the negative emotional baggage we are carrying.

This does not mean that I reject taking full advantage of traditional medical treatments. I researched thoroughly and was very grateful to follow a chemotherapy regimen. I believe that this chemo cured me of my physical symptoms of lymphoma, which is certainly not negligible. But I think we can truly *heal* by uncovering and resolving our outstanding emotional issues and thus change our thoughts.

My experience using the readings and methods of Claudia Rainville, and having an intensive therapy session with her, put me on the road to healing my lymphoma.

Of course, I also used the available Western medical treatments. But I do not believe that they would have been sufficient in the ongoing control of my disease, because I would not have resolved the underlying cause. Either I would have a recurrence of the lymphoma, or another form of illness.

My message therefore is about healing the emotions and thought patterns in order to heal the physical. It is clear to me that cleansing your thoughts and actions of negatively-charged emotions will improve both your daily quality of life as well as increase your chances of extending your life. Perhaps some are cured without going into the depth to which I refer, but I would not even consider taking such a chance.

There is a role played as a trigger by unhealthy habits such as smoking, but this does not explain why some three pack-a-day smokers do not die of lung cancer, and thousands who never smoked do.

LA PENSÉE MAGIQUE

There is a popular Quebec expression in French: *La pensée magique* or Magical Thinking.

It is generally used somewhat derisively, as if the person were extremely naïve, unworldly and living in La La Land.

It often crops up in discussions of politics and economics, implying that the individual should "get real."

It also appears frequently when human behaviour issues arise and it is felt that there is a lack of acceptance of the ugly side of human nature. It infers a Pollyannaish approach to a situation that is quite unsophisticated.

But, what if?

What if there is another way of thinking that does lead to magical results?

As Wayne Dyer outlines in his book, *The Power of Intention*, there does exist an alternative approach.

Our thoughts are all important in effecting what happens in our lives.

What we send out in thought energy is precisely what comes back to us. If I am unloving, that is returned to me and I wonder why the world is so full of such people. If I expect bad news, I shall receive it. If I am anxious and filled with worry, the world will appear to me in the same manner. Should I focus my thoughts on any form of lack in my life, this lack will not go away.

If, however, we look for goodness, are optimistic, seek and offer the best for others, and refrain from judgement, that is how our world will appear to us. The thinking itself is not magical, in the sense that it is readily available to all. But the results are.

My great challenge of course is in actually changing so that I think and live this way. But awareness is powerful, and it is the first step to achieving this.

I believe that the reason Claudia Rainville's therapeutic approach is so effective is because it, in fact, causes us to change our thought patterns (which have become our beliefs) related to a prior traumatic event in our lives. She initiates her discussion of this event by having us identify the emotions we felt at that moment. It is usually easier to identify *how* we felt rather than *what* we thought in an emotionally-charged situation.

But in reality, as I mentioned before, our emotions are formed by our thoughts. In changing our emotional perception, we are also changing our thoughts of that given situation.

With her method, my judgemental, critical, and guilt-laden thoughts were transformed into love, kindness, and forgiveness. I was led to understand the motivations and past traumas of the other who caused my pain.

This is where her approach leads directly to the message of Wayne Dyer's "intention."

He asks us to put aside the siren call of the ego and concentrate on kindness and compassion towards ourselves and others, no matter that we were "right" or felt we were treated badly by another.

Not easy to put into practice, given how we have lived our lives so far.

Individual needs and wants so often pre-empt consideration and compassion for others. We are taught to "stand up for ourselves," but, self-respect does not include the need to always believe we know the "truth" and the other is "wrong."

For me, kindness to others (and to ourselves) is the key to returning to and maintaining health, both physical and emotional. Of vital importance is the kindness to ourselves. My new behaviour is to try to treat myself as kindly as I would treat my best friend.

For about ten years now, I have believed that, if we are of sound mind, our personal happiness results directly from a choice we make. Quite simply, we can choose to be happy or not.

This is not another self-centered, highly individualistic way to live. Rather, we have full control over how we *react* to external events, not to the events themselves.

There is a fascinating book by Dr. David Hawkins called *Power vs Force*. He has developed and quantified what he calls a "Map of Consciousness." It represents a hierarchy of levels of consciousness (or spiritual growth) along with their concomitant emotions.

All of the negative emotions, such as shame, guilt, anger, fear, and pride fall into the self-destructive side. Only once we reach the level of courage, do we enter a positive, life-affirming context. For him, what we hold in our mind (our thoughts and beliefs) directly causes how we view the world, and therefore how the world will appear to us.

We have been "infected" by beliefs we unsuspectingly picked up out of our environment from a very early age. They are so ingrained that we do not even realize we have them, until we hold them up to the light. We can decide what thoughts we choose.

In his book *Healing and Recovery*, David Hawkins states that underlying every illness is a feeling of guilt that we must understand and address in order for healing to occur.

I find this fascinating, as Bernard had suggested to me a while ago to look into a feeling of guilt I had concerning my Mom. Now this really perplexed me for several weeks as my Mom and I were so close. But again, one day in a state of self-hypnosis with Nicole, my osteopath, I suddenly had the realization of what caused this guilt. This has allowed me to recognize, understand and eliminate it.

I do not ignore or forget the misery and suffering so prevalent in the world. But on a daily basis, the manner in which I choose to live and the thoughts I allow and nourish can at the very least bring kindness and joy to those I meet.

Let me share with you the gift that my friend Anik offered me: "Be curious and open-minded, be courageous, and trust your gut even when others do not."

And let me add:

Open your heart to the people around you and let them help and love you, while steadfastly maintaining your belief in yourself.

Keep or quickly regain your sense of humour.

Appreciate that there is always someone else who is having a worse day than you are, but also allow yourself to wallow in self-pity for very short periods. (After about one hour, I find this gets boring).

Keep faith in your hope.

Remember that to radiate happiness is the most powerful gift we can share with others and ourselves.

Watch your thoughts, for they become words
Watch your words for they become actions
Watch your actions for they become habits
Watch you habits for they become character
Watch your character for it becomes your destiny

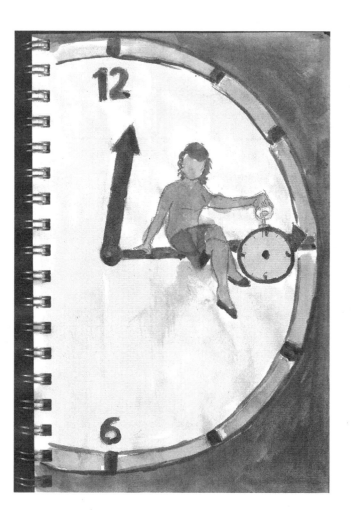

Acknowledgements

This chapter is both difficult and gratifying to write. Gratifying because it is so important to me to have the opportunity to thank the people who are responsible for this book's very existence. And difficult because I do not want anyone to feel unappreciated.

To begin, my book would most probably never have been written, if my wonderful friend, Anik, had not introduced me to Bernard Desgroppes, an amazing medium in Bordeaux, France. Merci Bernard for telling me that I was going to write a book that would be helpful to others facing health challenges. And had my publisher, Robin Philpot, not fortuitously decided to grant me the long-sought opportunity to be published, this book would have continued to languish in unread piles at various publishing houses throughout North America. For an unknown author to be published is somewhat miraculous. I am immensely grateful to you three.

Mon ami Jean-Pierre Dubreuil in Boston has provided the wonderful drawings in the book. Merci. Thanks to Michel Filion in Montreal for the evocative photo of me with my Havanese puppy.

Several of you have read different versions and shared support and helpful suggestions. Thanks Dana, Brigid, Cath, Diane, David, and Sylvie.

My family and friends have been my bulwark during these past ten years, with me at chemo sessions, feeding my body and soul, making me laugh and letting me cry. I cannot even imagine how I would have made it without you. To my sister Anne, Monique, Carole, Andrée, Mike, Robert, Michele, Laurie and my wonderful gang at Silver Islet, thank you all from the depths of my heart.

NOTABLE FICTION FROM BARAKA BOOKS

A Stab at Life, A Mystery Novel by Richard King

Things Worth Burying, A Novel by Matt Mayr

Exile Blues by Douglas Gary Freeman

Fog by Rana Bose

The Daughters' Story by Murielle Cyr

Yasmeen Haddad Loves Joanasi Maqaittik by Carolyn Marie Souaid

Vic City Express by Yannis Tsirbas (translated from the Greek by Fred A. Reed)

A Beckoning War by Matt Murphy

The Nickel Range Trilogy by Mick Lowe
   The Raids
   The Insatiable Maw
   Wintersong

AND FROM QC FICTION, AN IMPRINT OF BARAKA BOOKS

Songs for the Cold of Heart by Eric Dupont (translated by Peter McCambridge) 2018 Giller Finalist

The Little Fox of Mayerville by Éric Mathieu (translated by Peter McCambridge)

Prague by Maude Veilleux (translated by Aleshia Jensen & Aimée Wall)

In the End They Told Them All to Get Lost by Laurence Leduc-Primeau (translated by Natalia Hero)

NOTABLE NONFICTION

The Complete Muhammad Ali by Ishmael Reed

A Distinct Alien Race, The Untold Story of Franco-Americans by David Vermette

Through the Mill, Girls and Women in the Quebec Cotton Textile Industry, 1881-1951 by Gail Cuthbert Brandt

The Einstein File, The FBI's Secret War on the World's Most Famous Scientist by Fred Jerome

Montreal, City of Secrets, Confederate Operations in Montreal During the American Civil War by Barry Sheehy

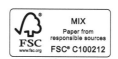